FOOD CRAVINGS

by Lisa Shock, B.Sc.
with
Robert Erdmann, Ph.D.

Shock, Lisa, 1953–
    Food cravings

ISBN 1–896817–03–3

    1. Compulsive eating. 2. Food preferences.
I. Erdmann, Robert, 1928–   II. Title.

RC552.C65S56 1998   616.85'26   C98–900268–3

Apple Publishing Company Ltd.
220 East 59th Avenue
Vancouver, British Columbia
Canada V5X 1X9
Tel (604) 214-6688 • Fax (604) 214-3566
Email: books@applepublishing.com

CONTENTS

INTRODUCTION

I first stumbled onto the cause (and cure) for food cravings while implementing several alternative medicinal methods to improve my health. I noticed for the first time in my life that I had no food cravings. It woke me up to the realization that these food cravings were **not normal**. Better yet, they could be stopped!

I have always been interested in food and food cravings. Even as a child I would go from one snack to another, first eating potato chips as I craved the salt and fat, then switching to dill pickles for a sour food, and then to chocolate for a sweet. I never got hungry. My stomach was always full, but no matter how full I was, I often craved something else. So I continued to eat until I was so bloated and I couldn't take another bite. In my ignorance I thought I was normal. Everyone else I knew also had food cravings, so I presumed the cravings were normal and unavoidable. I fostered the false impression that some people just have a stronger will power to control their cravings. Now I know better. All food cravings indicate chemical imbalances, and the more severe the imbalance the stronger the cravings. To control cravings all you need to do is identify the imbalance and correct it.

There have been many extensive research studies into the

physical nature of food cravings, but little practical help for the average consumer. Most of the advice that has been published advises using behavior modification to control cravings. The results with these methods are highly variable and often stressful. Why fight cravings? There is an alternative. You can learn from your craving. It is telling you exactly what is wrong. By learning the language of our body, and how to correctly interpret what these cravings really mean we can work with our body to restore balance. Like magic the craving just goes away, often in seconds.

CHAPTER 1

CRAVINGS

According to surveys, food cravings plague 97% of women and 68% of men. They can be the urge for chocolate, french fries, potato chips, salty, sour, buttery, fried foods, pizza, ice cream, beer, wine, tobacco, or a myriad of foods. Cravings can even be more bizarre, with urges for dirt, minerals and other non-food items. Someone who has never had strong cravings may think the urge is just an indication of poor self control, but those of us with cravings know better.

Cravings have always existed as they are survival mechanisms. Man has always had the instinct to crave certain foods while avoiding others. Sweet cravings encourage consumption of fruits and vegetables. These naturally occurring sweet foods, are usually high in food value. The high carbohydrate content of fruits and vegetables are balanced with vitamins and minerals essential for health. Fats are also instinctively craved. Rich sources of fat normally accompany high protein foods, that are also high in many essential nutrients. This instinct worked well in man's early history to preserve life by encouraging consumption of healthy foods. Poisonous plants usually taste bitter. The aversion to bitter foods helps us to avoid these poisons.

The problems started when food became abundant, and quality diminished. Modern farming with chemicals left soils depleted of nutrients, and the plants grown on those soils, deficient. Processing and refining removed more nutrient value, and even fresh organic foods lost much of their value from cooking or storage. The instinct to eat sweet or fatty foods still exists, but many of these foods have become so depleted that eventually nutritional deficiencies occur.

Salt cravings are also common. They occur primarily in plant-eating animals. A diet high in plants is often too low in salt, stimulating cravings. Easy access to salt by people with chemical imbalances can lead to excessive consumption of these foods. In an attempt to improve health, some people have eliminated salt from their diet, but it is a vital nutrient that is essential to good health. The cravings for salt exist for a very good reason and should not be ignored. No farmer in his right mind would eliminate the salt blocks in his cattle pasture. Free access to salt is essential for his animals' health and his economic success. Overconsumption of salt is not normally an issue for the farmer. When the animal is healthy it will only consume appropriate amounts of salt. People can also learn from this example. In a state of health we will regulate our salt intake as our taste dictates to maintain health. It is only when our health deteriorates that cravings can take over and further destroy health unless steps are taken to reverse the cravings.

Chemical imbalances trigger food cravings. Understanding the cues to these cravings allows an intelligent approach to eliminating them. Our body and mind work hard to keep us healthy and preserve life. Food cravings are just a misguided attempt to restore balance. When our body chemistry is out of balance, the mind and body will respond by producing chemicals that alter behavior. These brain chemicals then trigger a craving. Scientists have identified several of these chemicals, classified as neuropeptides. The neuropeptide Y causes carbohydrate cravings. The neuropeptide galanin causes fat cravings. There are probably another 25 or 30 more neuropeptides waiting to be identified that also control cravings. Hormones (insulin, estrogen and progesterone) also affect brain chemistry and can intensify cravings.

Sometimes the craving has a psychological component, a smell, or a thought can trigger the craving. Many people get cravings while watching TV commercials. This is due to past behavior and conditioning, but it too can be effectively stopped. Smell can 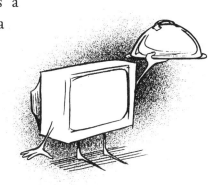 be the most powerful stimulus both to start and stop a craving, and is one of the "triggers" you can use to your benefit once you learn how.

The methods in this book can give you the assistance to break the cycle of compulsive eating. You can still enjoy your favorite foods, but now you can choose when and what to eat. I have found new delight in eating the foods I once craved. Now that I eat them for sheer enjoyment, the flavors are savored that much more. The craving had compelled me to eat without the enjoyment, stuffing the food down but not really enjoying it. It is true that I now eat them less frequently since the cravings are gone, but I never miss them.

We are all individuals with different metabolisms, and

different nutritional needs. As you apply these techniques to eliminate your food cravings you will notice where you get the best results. The discovery of which technique works best for you will empower you to take control of your appetite. Be sure to keep notes on what works best for you, so that if the cravings return you will know the fastest way to quickly eliminate it. Some of the material in this book may be too technical (or not technical enough as the case may be) to suit you. I have attempted to write this book at a level that will be the most useful to the greatest number of people.

CHAPTER 2

COMPULSIVE EATING

STRESS, BOREDOM, LONELINESS OR ANGER

This chapter deals with general food cravings, when there is a desire to eat anything. The opposite of eating is fasting. In my opinion eating is necessary to sustain life. Fasting can be very dangerous to your health, and should only be attempted with a doctor's supervision. Medically supervised fasting programs use juices with fiber and absorbent additives. In addition, nutritional supplements suitable to individual needs are incorporated into the program, but still require planning and monitoring.

The techniques in this book can be useful to people that want to cut back on their eating because they have been consuming excessive calories. Actual hunger is a call to eat, and ignoring it can result in numerous health problems, the first of which is usually low blood sugar levels. These low blood sugar levels result in weakness and fatigue. Eventually resulting in the breakdown of proteins to manufacture the glucose vital to brain function. The final consequences are often food cravings leading to a food binge.

If you've ever been "stressed out" you may have been compelled to start munching. Stress can induce compulsive overeating. Eating calms frayed nerves. You don't need to pig out. Instead, identify your symptoms and take the appropriate supplement or action.

IRRITABILITY, ANGER AND STRESS

If you eat when irritable, angry or just stressed out, perhaps you are just trying to calm your nerves. Meditation or exercise are the most common methods recommended to reduce stress. If your schedule or personality is not suited to these methods, there are other options. You can try a blend of nutritional supplements that have been shown to be useful in a variety of clinical malaises including: allergies, asthma, migraine headaches, pain, obsessive-compulsive behavior, manic depressive problems, tremor control, insomnia, and other health problems. Most people report the **calming effect** occurs within minutes.

Try these supplements:

Histamine	Glycine
Taurine	Inositol
Thiamine	Riboflavin
Pyridoxine	Vitamin C
Calcium	Niacinamide

Bio-Science (a nutritional supplement supplier) has put these all together in a capsule called **"Calma Complex"** (see sources). I have used these capsules freely to calm frayed nerves, sometimes using 6 at a time to get fast results. Taking the individual components will also work for those with the time to experiment at getting the most effective dosage for their individual needs.

Other calming nutrients you can try are:
GABA (gamma-aminobutyric acid)

Vitamin B6

Magnesium

The most effective calming nutrient is **tryptophan**, an essential amino acid. The best food source is **Spirulina**. You'll need digestive enzymes to free up the tryptophan. "**Bio-Rest**", another Bio-Science product, is a source of Spirulina combined with digestive enzymes that works well as a source of tryptophan.

SADNESS, LONELINESS, DEPRESSION AND APATHY

Low levels of certain brain stimulants can change your moods, resulting in feelings of sadness, loneliness or boredom. This is especially noticeable in the morning. Do you have trouble getting up in the morning? Are you tired and sleepy for an hour or more in the morning? Supplemental amino acids can provide the building blocks to boost these brain stimulants. The amino acids: **phenylalanine, glutamine, tyrosine, or pyro-glutamic acid** can all act as stimulants. Take them in the morning before you eat. One or two grams work for most people, but can also increase blood pressure. If you have high blood pressure you will need a doctor's advice before taking these amino acids. Another product that helps many in the morning is **DHEA**. DHEA is used by the body to make hormones, and if your system is low on DHEA, it may not be making enough hormones to function at full capacity. Most experts recommend taking DHEA in the morning, however, a few people get better results by taking it at night. See what works best for you. Blood tests are the only accurate way to determine the optimum dose of DHEA. Most people over the age of 40 respond to doses of 10–200mg.

Herbs can also calm frayed nerves. The best calming herbs are:
Passion Flower   Primula Officinalis

Milder calming herbs include:
Valerian   Lobelia
Skullcap   Red Clover
Chamomile   Catnip
Hops

Vitamins and minerals can help reduce stress.
Take extra when you're feeling stressed out.
Especially important are the B vitamins:
Inositol   Niacin
Pyridoxine   Riboflavin
Thiamine

These anti-oxidants are also important:
Vitamin E   Vitamin D
Vitamin C   Lipoic Acid

Minerals that support your nerves include:
Calcium   Iodine
Iron   Magnesium
Phosphorus   Potassium
Silicon   Sodium

Excellent essential oils that can also calm you include
sandalwood and **jasmine** as well as **rose**.

CHAPTER 3

CARBOHYDRATE CRAVINGS—STARCHES

Carbohydrates may be separated into starches and sweets, but the truth is these cravings often overlap. Be sure to read both sections, then try the one that you think most accurately fits your craving. If you aren't getting good results, try suggestions from the other section.

Low brain levels of serotonin (be patient—I will explain what this is in more detail) is the most common cause of carbohydrate cravings, and along with low blood sugar accounts for almost all these cravings. The difference is hard to distinguish, but low serotonin usually causes cravings for pasta, bread, potatoes and starches, while low blood sugar may trigger cravings for sweets. This is not a strict rule so any craving for starchy or sweet foods should be examined for both.

Mineral deficiencies can further complicate these cravings. Chromium deficiency is perhaps the best known mineral that affects blood sugar levels. Undiagnosed diseases in chronic subclinical states can also trigger these cravings. Hepatitis, liver cirrhosis, parasites, kidney failure, cancer, diabetes, and several hormone disorders are states that affect taste, and increase the desire for sweeter and sweeter foods. Deficiencies of B12, vitamin A, and niacin as well as numerous drugs, antihistamines, ·antibiotics, cancer drugs, cholesterol medicine, and anaesthesia can also lead to carbohydrate cravings. Identifying and eliminating these causes goes a long way towards eliminating the physical craving.

Before we get too far into the actual brain chemistry I must also mention another brain chemical that plays a role in cravings. Sweet sensations on the tongue increase the brain chemicals called endorphins. Endorphins are mood elevators and pain relievers. The desire for sweet tastes, and the endorphins they produce can lead to "sweet tooth". Before modern farming, the original sweet food was fresh tree ripened fruit, and vine ripened vegetables, grown on rich organic soils. These were a potent source of vitamins, minerals, enzymes, fiber and nutrients. These healthy sweet foods restored balance and improved nutritional status of the individual. The endorphins served to reinforce this good behavior. Today's empty calories fail in the long run because they contain carbohydrates without the essential vitamins, minerals enzymes, and amino acids. If endorphins can make us feel good or just feel better when we feel bad then anything that stimulates endorphins like eating sweets is remembered and repeated. The brain stores up memories of which foods work best to relieve pain, elevate mood, and effectively alter brain chemistry. More about endorphins later, first let us look at the basic underlying brain chemistry that most commonly triggers carbohydrate cravings.

LOW SEROTONIN
Eating carbohydrates brings about changes in the brain chemicals, resulting in increased brain serotonin. Serotonin is a vital brain chemical and when it drops the brain produces

another chemical called neuropeptide Y that causes the food craving for carbohydrates. When carbohydrates are consumed, the first noticeable effect is an increase in blood sugar levels. This stimulates your metabolism and increases energy levels, heat is generated and body temperature increases, (a very useful feature for preventing hypothermia in cold environments.) Something else that happens is the increased blood sugar causes a decrease in almost all the blood amino acid levels, the building blocks of protein. Only one amino acid escapes this decrease and the level of tryptophan is actually increased. In the brain this now abundant tryptophan is converted to serotonin. Thus the increased blood level of tryptophan restores brain serotonin. But where does the blood get this tryptophan? The food you ate was carbohydrate, and thus low or totally void of tryptophan. The only place you can draw tryptophan from is your precious body reserves, mostly bound up in proteins. Humans lack the ability to manufacture tryptophan leaving only one method left to restore your reserves and that is to eventually eat food containing tryptophan. That is the only way to replenish your supplies. Eating carbohydrates only allows the tryptophan you already have stored to be released and converted to serotonin. Once the serotonin level rises in the brain, it calms, relaxes and eventually makes you sleepy if levels get high enough. Most people can relate to this sleep sensation after a large meal, especially if high in carbohydrates. Unfortunately eating refined carbohydrates such as chocolate, sweets, etc., ultimately aggravates the chemical imbalance. The tryptophan supply becomes more depleted, forcing the breakdown of proteins to supply tryptophan. The "high" from the endorphins in the brain continues to reinforce this faulty eating habit. The increased imbalance actually due to tryptophan deficiency in diet, only causes a stronger craving, and the cycle becomes worse.

The entire cycle looks something like this:

1. Insufficient tryptophan in the diet eventually leads to low levels in the brain.

2. Insufficient tryptophan in the brain means not enough serotonin is produced since serotonin is made from tryptophan.

3. Low brain serotonin triggers the brain to produce neuropeptide Y.

4. Neuropeptide Y induces carbohydrate cravings.

5. Eating the high carbohydrate food causes tryptophan to be increased from your body stores of proteins and other competing amino acids to be decreased. Thus brain levels of tryptophan increase.

6. Increased tryptophan leads to increased serotonin, thus solving the crises for your brain. If enough serotonin is produced, a warm sleepy sensation may follow.

7. The carbohydrate food didn't supply the tryptophan, instead it was supplied from your protein reserves, leaving them even more depleted. Unless restored by the diet the cycle will repeat once again.

8. High blood sugar levels from eating the carbohydrates stimulates insulin that pushes the sugars into your cells to be stored as fat. Once blood sugars are reduced the cycle repeats unless tryptophan is supplied by the diet.

All is not lost; the cycle can be broken and balance restored, but not by eating the empty carbohydrates you crave, instead, by understanding the true causes and thus treating them with appropriate foods, the brain chemistry balance can be restored.

Most sweets today are often empty calories. Even today, fruits, vegetables and grains contain just a shadow of the nutrients they once had. Fertilizers and poor soils have left them depleted, and processing and storage only exacerbate the problem. After eating devitalized food the chemical imbalance becomes worse, creating even stronger cravings. The initial relief from eating the carbohydrate is short lived and as soon as the high insulin pushes the blood sugar levels down the craving for sweets returns.

You can put this information to use whenever you have a carbohydrate craving, by recognizing the craving as serotonin depletion that can be restored only with the amino acid tryptophan, vitamins and minerals necessary for assimilation and conversion to serotonin.

HORMONE INFLUENCES

Chemical imbalances leading to low serotonin can also be triggered by excessive estrogen, progesterone, or other hormone levels. Many women find their cravings diminishing at the onset of menopause when these hormones decline, and conversely many pregnant women find their cravings increase during pregnancy and premenstrually when these hormones increase. The hormones don't cause the cravings, the chemical imbalance does. The hormones only make the problem worse. Normalizing high hormone levels is essential to good health and will diminish the cravings. The dietary changes that decrease cravings also go a long way to normalizing hormone levels. The body works together as one with each part affected by all the others. It is difficult and ill advised to try and lower your hormones artificially. While you will be affected by your hormones don't let high levels bother you. Just be aware of the influence and be alert to times when you will be more susceptible to food cravings. The real solution will be in reversing these cravings. You may even find the hormone levels returning to a more normal level after several months of controlling cravings. This can be attributed to healthier overall chemistry balance.

Low serotonin has also been found with:

Depression	Suicide
Anorexia	Alcoholism
Manic depressive disorder	Agoraphobia
Panic disorder	Impulsiveness
Kleptomania	Food binging
Anxiety	Poor memory
Insomnia	Apathy

All these problems can potentially benefit from utilizing the suggestions to increase serotonin. Some people even go so far as to suggest the above problems can be cured by restoring serotonin.

LOW SEROTONIN—STARCH CRAVINGS

When a carbohydrate craving strikes, stop it in its tracks! Then work on a long-term solution to stop cravings before they strike by balancing your body chemistry.

STEP ONE

Immediately eat some high protein food. Even just a few bites can often stop a carbohydrate craving in seconds. Some suggestions of high protein foods (with high tryptophan content) are:

1. Blue-green algae, especially Spirulina
2. Brewers yeast (1 oz.)
3. Soybeans (1/2 cup)
4. Cottage cheese (1/2 cup)
5. Pumpkin seeds (1/2 cup)
6. Watermelon seeds (dried, 1/2 cup)
7. Amino acid supplement: the amino acid tryptophan (1-5 grams)

For meat eaters try:

1. An egg
2. Chicken liver (3 oz.)
3. Turkey (3 oz.)
4. Chicken (3 oz.)
5. Tuna, canned in water

If a tryptophan supplement is available, it is the number one treatment. Otherwise you'll have to get it from complex foods. For convenience there is one nutritional product that is high in tryptophan from natural sources. The product is called "Bio-Rest", it is a combination of the richest food source of tryptophan (Spirulina) with digestive enzymes to free up the tryptophan, and co-factors to enhance conversion to serotonin. *(See Sources for where to obtain this product or be sure to take extra enzymes with your Spirulina.)*

STEP TWO

Drink two large glasses of **Water**. Dehydration to some extent is common with most chemical imbalances. Water dilutes the chemical imbalance and reverses the dehydration. This assists the body in restoring harmony.

STEP THREE

Stress also lowers serotonin levels. If the above nutrients are not available, try these methods until you can get some. To reduce stress try listening to some pleasant classical music. Music has long been known to relieve stress. If music is unavailable try singing something uplifting and joyful. Many religious, patriotic, and holiday songs are useful. If all else fails, try humming vowels, AEIOU. Start with A, hum it as low as possible, taking a full long breath to slowly hum A..., now repeat with E..., etc. When done start over gradually raising the pitch with each series. Rest for a moment when done.

STEP FOUR

Increase serotonin by:
1. Exercising
2. Getting outside in the sunlight
3. Using a negative ion generator
4. Stand in a shower

Negative ions increase serotonin and water produces negative ions also, that's why showers, waterfalls and oceans feel so great.

CHAPTER 4

SUGAR CRAVINGS

Low blood sugar levels can also trigger cravings for sweets. Eating something sweet or starchy will increase blood sugar temporarily. A small meal is good at reversing low blood sugar, but a large one will boomerang. Overeating results in too high of blood sugar forcing the pancreas to respond by making insulin. The insulin then works to lower blood sugar. This creates a cycle where sweets are craved, then eaten, you feel good followed by sleepiness. The craving cycle starts all over again.

Sometimes the body loses its ability to regulate blood sugar levels resulting in disease. Diabetics exhaust their pancreas and it doesn't produce enough insulin. Hypoglycemics are in the process of wearing out their pancreas, as it overproduces insulin. People fasting or just skipping meals are also risking low blood sugar levels. Skipping meals is probably the most common cause of food cravings. Within reason, *never* again skip a meal.

Eating small frequent meals will keep blood sugar levels more stable and even. This approach is commonly known as "grazing."

By eating a small quantity (usually about 1/2 to 1 cup food) every 90 minutes, the stomach is kept working, slowly releasing nutrients. Only healthy food, such as fresh vegetables, whole fruits, complex grains, sprouts and flax oil should be consumed. It is an effective diet program for weight loss and pancreatic dysfunction. It will stabilize blood sugar, but only if followed precisely. Too often we become busy and we eat "junk food", or else forget to eat at the prescribed time. The blood sugar drops and hunger triggers a craving. This is a tricky diet, but workable for those with the ability to stick to strict schedules.

You will need a fully functional pancreas and basic good eating habits to eliminate sweet cravings permanently. To stop them temporarily try the following methods.

TO STOP SUGAR CRAVINGS

STEP ONE

If you are suffering from low blood sugar, you must do something to increase the blood sugar level, as quickly and safely as possible. If the problem has escalated to weakness and a shaky feeling, you need food immediately. Most severe hypoglycemics feel so bad that they don't even want to eat anything. This just increases symptoms.

To help restore blood sugar levels, take:
    4 L-Cysteine capsules (500 mg)
    1 Vitamin C pill (1000 mg)
    1 Vitamin B1 (100 mg)

Eat about 4 oz. of complex carbohydrates. I like a handful of **wheat sprouts.** Eat some **protein,** the same as step one for starch cravings. Keep a supply of **Spirulina** tablets or capsules on hand. Take 6 capsules. They have minerals, vitamins and protein that can often stop cravings in their tracks. Follow with a large glass of water. Be sure to rest 30 minutes while you are getting the blood sugar levels back to normal.

STEP TWO

Nutritional yeast can sometimes help. Take a large spoonful with a glass of milk or juice.

STEP THREE

If you are craving sweets be sure to try the herb from India, **Gymnema sylvestre.** It has been shown to decrease the craving for sweets for several hours after consumption of the leaves. It has also been used to normalize blood lipids (triglycerides and cholesterol), and enhance insulin production in diabetics. Diabetes is a complex disease, and should only be treated under a doctor's supervision. A complete program using this herb, diet, and other nutritional supplements has been used to help many diabetics, but only under a doctor's supervision.

STEP FOUR

Fool your taste buds! By fooling your taste buds you can get the brain to release endorphins. Put something in your mouth that tastes sweet but won't cause the problems that sugar does. I like **stevia extract** as a sweetener, or vegetable **glycerine** in small amounts. I do NOT use Aspartame (Nutra-Sweet™). There are too many questions regarding the safety of Aspartame, and it may also cause weight gain and increased appetite in some people.

STEP FIVE

Try a **zinc lozenge.** I use a pleasant tasting zinc lozenge that slowly dissolves on my tongue. Zinc is probably the most common mineral deficiency associated with low blood sugar and easy to correct.

STEP SIX

If you are still having problems with sweet cravings you may need another of the following supplements. You will have to experiment with these supplements unless you go to the expense of a nutritional testing. I have listed several supplements. Some work fast at controlling cravings but some take time, so be consistent if you want lasting results. Poor regulation of blood sugar levels can sometimes improve with **chromium** supplements, but only if chromium is lacking. Mineral and vitamin supplements can often assist in normalizing body chemistry, requiring individual assessment to be truly effective. Without testing you are just guessing at mineral and vitamin deficiencies. To be safe you should take a balanced multiple supplement. Just taking one mineral or vitamin can actually cause further imbalance in others.

Mineral deficiencies associated with sugar craving include:

Magnesium	Calcium
Chromium	Zinc
Iron	Copper
Manganese	Vanadium
Selenium	

Vitamins associated with sugar cravings are primarily the **B vitamins.** Taking high dose multiple B vitamins can often help. Chewing the vitamin pills allows better absorption and may actually be essential in some people. B vitamins are water soluble and high doses will be quickly excreted in the urine if taken in excess of body needs. Only extreme high doses over long periods of time can result in side effects from overdosing. Dosages currently available as B100 type pills contain either 100 mg or 100 mcg of all B vitamins. These amounts are quite safe even for prolonged periods. High dose side effects are not usually a problem until the dose approaches 20 times this amount, and is maintained for weeks or months. The problem of establishing optimum vitamin dosages occurs due to individual variation, some people actually require 1500 mg B6 daily, a dose that might eventually be toxic to another individual. This is where the assistance of a naturopath, or orthomolecular nutritionist can be essential in individualizing dosages. For most average folks taking one of those "B 100" pills is often adequate.

Vitamins known to be associated with blood sugar level regulation:

Niacin	Niacinamide
Biotin	B1 – thiamine
B2 – riboflavin	B6 – pyridoxine HCL
B5 – pantothenic acid	Folic acid
B12	Vitamin C
Vitamin E	Vitamin D

Amino acids are also important in regulating blood sugar levels. Extra supplemental sources of **l-Carnitine & Glutamic acid** are useful in regulating blood sugar.

Herbs can be incorporated into a program to regulate blood sugar. The above mentioned herb **gymnema** is the most powerful, but leaf extracts from **zyziphus jujube** are also effective. Weaker herbs that have a more generalized tonic effect on blood sugar regulation include:

Dandelion	Juniper and Cedar berries
Licorice	Safflower

to a lesser extent:

Alfalfa	Bee Pollen
Blue Cohosh	Black Cohosh
Catnip	Chlorophyll

Don Quai	Hawthorn
Horseradish	Kelp
Lobelia	Marshmallow
Skullcap	Valerian

The herb to avoid if you suffer from hypoglycemia is **golden seal** as it can make your condition worse.

CHAPTER 5

SALT CRAVINGS

Salt which is sodium chloride is essential for life. We instinctively crave salt to replenish the natural losses that constantly occur. Salt craving may be expressed as a craving for pretzels, bacon, ham, pickles, or any salty food. Read the labels to see which products have lots of added salt. The urge for something salty is often combined with other urges. The salt urge may not be apparent to you, instead you may think what you want is potato chips. If the food you crave has lots of salt, (and almost all processed foods do have lots of salt,) you must first determine if you crave salt or something else in the food. You may find that you crave both salt and fat, or salt, fat and starch, or any other combination. Most people get plenty of salt in their diet, but not enough potassium. Potassium and sodium (from salt) are closely related. Potassium often gets overlooked as a potential problem in salt cravings and if you actually do crave salt, you may need potassium and/or sodium. The first step is to determine if you crave the salt or something else in the food.

Salt is a flavor enhancer thus it can make foods taste sweeter. This is probably why it is so commonly used. Salt is found in processed foods, and candy, including chocolate. There are also certain health conditions and prescription drug side effects that cause salt and sugar cravings.

When salt becomes dangerously depleted you can die. Heat exhaustion is sometimes attributed to low salt levels. Even mild exercise in a hot environment can increase salt losses through perspiration. To save salt or fluids due to other physical problem, the body stops sweating, and the person overheats. If salt levels are dangerously low, then salt will take on a sweet taste, indicating salt is dangerously depleted. People that restrict their salt intake or those that sweat excessively are prone to salt deficiency.

Several illnesses and medications can cause salt and potassium problems. If you constantly crave salt your doctor should be made aware of this problem. If the craving is occasional and you are in good health without any medical problems or taking medications then you should be sure to consult your doctor about any health problems or concerns before attempting to implement any of the following suggestions.

Low adrenal function is a common, but often hidden condition that can lead to excessive salt losses. When the adrenal glands are not working properly, excessive sodium can be lost in the urine. Many people have low adrenal function from poor nutrition and excessive stress. This state is often associated with orthostatic hypotension. Orthostatic hypotension means that your blood pressure drops when you sit or stand up quickly. It is just a technical term to describe a symptom. A simple test for orthostatic hypotension is to lie down for a few minutes, then stand up quickly! Don't jump up —just stand up. Did you get light-headed or dizzy? How about any vision problems? If you answered yes, you probably suffer from orthostatic hypotension, and adrenal fatigue. If you really want to see how severe the problem is, you'll need someone trained to measure blood pressure. Take your blood pressure while lying down, then sit up and take it again, then stand and take it again. In a normal person the difference in blood pressure readings will increase 4 to 10 mmHg. as you rise. Any readings that drop or fail to increase at least 4 points for each change in position indicate orthostatic hypotension, and indicate adrenal fatigue. This method to determine adrenal function is called the Ragland Effect and has been used for over 50 years, mostly by alternative medicine doctors to determine low adrenal function.

Low adrenal function can also affect your nerve function. This can be tested using a mirror and flashlight. While looking at your pupil in the mirror, shine the flashlight in your eye. Hold the flashlight about 6 inches from the eye, or at a comfortable distance depending on the strength of the light. The pupil should contract and stay contracted as long as the light is directed toward it. If you get dilation, or initial contraction followed by dilation, it indicates adrenal problems that need to be addressed. Those tests were simple and painless but if you now suspect low adrenal function, you should also expect excessive sodium losses in the urine. As the sodium becomes depleted, dehydration and excessive urine production also occur, increasing the need for both salt and water in the diet. You also need to address the low adrenal problem with nutritional support and dietary changes. Try taking daily:

Vitamin C: 5000mg

B complex (100 high potency)

Pantothenic acid: 500–2000mg

Malic acid

Magnesium: dose to effect

Adrenal supplements: dose to effect

DHEA: 50–200mg
Nutritional testing would help

You may also have a problem tasting the salt in your food. If your taste for salt is impaired, your brain might think "this food needs salt", but actually it has ample salt. Salt taste buds become saturated from high salt foods, and you lose the ability to fully taste the salt in your food. The more you salt your food, the more you lose the ability to taste the salt. When this occurs a brief respite from salt is all that is needed to restore salt-tasting ability.

Next test for iodine deficiency. Salt and iodine are naturally found together in many foods, especially seafoods. Kelp and seaweed are a wonderful source of many trace minerals, including iodine. You can perform a simple screening test by applying a small amount of weak iodine solution to your skin, just before retiring. In the morning check the color of the iodine spot. If it is significantly lighter, or gone, this indicates you are readily absorbing iodine. The more your body needs iodine, the more it absorbs it. Once you have reached the point where you don't require additional iodine, your skin will slow the absorption. Of course it is possible to overdo iodine, so you'll need to monitor the skin test and consume safe amounts. Natural foods like kelp and seaweed are the safest way to increase iodine and other trace minerals in the diet.

Once you have eliminated the potential causes of salt cravings listed thus far, two possible causes of salt cravings remain: low sodium or low potassium. The following taste test can indicate these deficiencies but you will need to get a solution of potassium phosphorus called "Chem.test 1" from Bio-Science (*see sources*) to test your potassium needs:

1. Mix 1 tsp. salt in 8 oz. water and taste.

2. If the salt solution tastes good, mild, or sweet you need sodium. If it tastes bad, too salty, or awful you don't need sodium. To get more sodium in your diet you should eat salt with your food and drink lots of water.

3. Mix 13 drops of Chem.test 1 potassium phosphorus solution (see sources), in 8 oz. of water, and taste.

4. If the Chem.test 1 solution tastes good, mild, or OK, you need potassium. If it tastes bad, or awful you don't need potassium. To get more potassium in your diet, try and eat more vegetables, and use potassium chloride as a salt substitute.

5. To get more of both potassium and sodium use a "little salt" (half potassium chloride and half sodium chloride) liberally on your food and drink lots of water.

6. To get more sodium in your diet just add more salt.

Extensive testing of blood, and urine can reveal the cause of salt cravings, but are more expensive than these simple taste tests. If you don't want to bother with taste tests, that's OK. Just go on to the steps that follow.

If you are in good health, and have no dietary restrictions (check with your doctor) you can take the following steps when a salt craving strikes.

TO STOP A SALT CRAVING

STEP ONE
Take a cracker, or slice of cucumber, or tomato, or something else you like to eat with salt. Dump some "lite salt" onto the

cracker or other item. About 1/2 tsp. will usually do it. Now eat up. Follow with a large glass of water. If one dose helps, but you still crave salt, wait a little while and try a second dose. Some people may need a little extra, depending on their body chemistry. If you can not eat salt due to special dietary restrictions, you can try plain potassium chloride.

STEP TWO
If you still have a craving, it may be for something other than the salt. If the food is rich in fat, carbohydrates, or is meat, go to that section. Mineral deficiencies should also be considered. Add kelp or seaweed to your diet on a regular basis or take a kelp supplement.

CHAPTER 6

FAT CRAVINGS

French fries, potato chips, butter, sour cream, margarine, fried food, cheese (it's often loaded with fat), bacon, ham, and fatty meats can all be part of a FAT craving. Fat gives food flavor and improves texture. The brain releases endorphins to reward us for eating fat, and creates chemical triggers to induce fat cravings when essential fatty acids are too low. Some dietary fat is essential for life. Your body requires several nutrients from foods that it can not make on its own. Vitamins, minerals, and certain amino acids are well known for their essential role in nutrition. What is commonly overlooked in diets are the essential fatty acids. While we can make many fats, and that is how we store excess calories, there are a few fats that we can not make. We need these essential Omega -3 and Omega -6 fatty acids. They are vital for every cell in our body, and we must get them from food, we can not make them. Most foods have virtually none, or only trace amounts of these essential fatty acids. There are only a few good food sources. Flax oil and olive oil combined half and half, make about the best food source you can find.

Oils must be kept refrigerated and used up within a few months of purchase, to retain top quality. Light, heat, and oxygen all destroy these essential oils, producing toxic trans-fatty acids. A deficiency of these essential fatty acids is often the source of a fat craving. Protein (or the amino acid 1-cysteine), inositol, and bile are essential to proper absorption of these vital fats. Flax oil is especially vulnerable to the ravages of heat, light and oxygen. It must be processed at cold temperatures, without oxygen. This is accomplished only with specialized equipment and oxygen free chambers. I recommend Barlean's Organic Flax Oil, available in most health food stores or by mail order. Its mild nutty taste makes it my favorite oil for use in salad dressings. It is processed with the best technology available resulting in a product with superior taste and nutrients.

WHEN A FAT CRAVING STRIKES

STEP ONE
Take all of the following:
1. One or two tablespoons **flax oil,**
   or flax mixed with **olive oil** 50–50.
2. 500–2000mg **l-Cysteine**
3. 1 tablespoon **lemon juice**
4. 1 **inositol** capsule

STEP TWO
If the above doesn't work, try a tablespoon of **cod liver oil.** The vitamins and co-factors it contains often correct the problem. It comes in several flavors that mask the fish taste.

STEP THREE
If you have trouble digesting and absorbing fat, add the following to step one:
1. Take several **lipase enzymes** along with fat.

2. Take a supplement containing **bile salts**
   (Beta-Plus for example, see *Sources*).

STEP FOUR

If you have light colored stools, no problem with constipation, and suffer from gas, bloating or a history of gall bladder attacks, then you may need to stimulate the liver and bile. With each meal take:

1. Beet powder
2. Taurine
3. Pancrealipase
4. Vitamin C
5. Iodine supplement
6. Phosphatidylcholine
7. B Vitamins, with extra B6 phosphate
8. Magnesium

STEP FIVE

Sunshine has been called an "activator" of fats. Winter, with its lower levels of sunshine, often increases the craving for fats. This naturally results in more body fat to increase survival in primitive conditions where food shortages occurred in late winter and spring. With ample year-round food we don't need this extra body fat, but the lack of sunshine still creates the craving. Get out in the sun or get some high intensity lighting.

Natural sunshine has a healthy spectrum of wavelengths that are ideal. High intensity lighting falls far short of sunshine but will be of some benefit. Some people claim full spectrum lighting products are superior to other artificial lights. They usually cost up to 15 times more than regular light bulbs. The full spectrum may be beneficial for certain conditions, however the research on cravings showed the benefit was more a function of the intensity. The more light the better, regardless of the source.

Sunlight has the greatest intensity and thus it is preferred. If your finances are such that you can afford the high cost of full spectrum, it may provide a slightly better light source, but it can never completely duplicate the benefits of natural sunlight.

STEP SIX
Parasite problems are common with fat cravings. Especially when fat and proteins are both craved. Help from a doctor, or a health professional may be required to identify and treat parasite problems.

STEP SEVEN
Butter cravings could be a way for the body to get butyric acid. Certain butter fats are changed by intestinal bacteria into butyric acid, which aids beneficial bacteria (the acidophilus family) in adhering to the intestinal wall. Butyric acid supplements have been used for this purpose, as a supplement to treat candida, colitis, diverticulitis, and other intestinal diseases. If you suspect this problem, a short trial with butyric acid supplements, and acidophilus cultures could be useful. Stool tests can also determine if you require this supplement.

STEP EIGHT
Release endorphins *(see section on endorphins)*.

CHAPTER 7

CHOCOLATE

Chocolate is such a commonly craved food that I listed it separately. Actually chocolate cravings can be traced to chocolate's components which are primarily sugar, magnesium, salt, fat, amines, and caffeine.

SUGAR
Chocolate is high in sugar and low blood sugar levels may trigger a craving.

MAGNESIUM
Chocolate is high in magnesium and some researchers speculate up to 95% of the population may have some magnesium deficiency. A low magnesium level may trigger chocolate craving.

SALT
Chocolate has salt to enhance flavor.

ENDORPHINS
Chocolate stimulates endorphins in the brain and these pleasure chemicals are addictive and can induce cravings. Some people (especially women) rush out and eat chocolate when they are sad. Women suffer more from sad and unhappy feelings, their brains show much more activity when sad,

resulting in intense emotional pain. Emotional pain can be devastating and chocolate is craved to ease the suffering. Once you learn how to stimulate these endorphins in healthy ways you get relief without chocolate.

FAT
Chocolate is also high in fats which are a common craving.

AMINES
Chocolate is full of amines. Amines are a large group of organic compounds that our body utilizes for dozens of functions. In order to be classified as an amine, all that is required is that the molecule have an amine group. Most, but not all, of these chemicals, have a name that ends in "amine". There are some good amines that your body makes and uses to maintain health like serotonin and dopamine, and some "bad" amines that are toxic. Unfortunately the amines in chocolate are the "bad or toxic" kind. Toxic amines cause high blood pressure, headaches, and have been implicated in strokes. To get rid of the "bad or toxic" amines our body makes an enzyme to break them down. This enzyme monoamine oxidase, is called MAO for short. When your toxic amines get high, your body responds by increasing MAO levels. These high MAO levels ultimately lower your "good" amines also, including serotonin. Low serotonin then leads to further cravings. Hormones increase MAO activity, resulting in "premenstrual cravings" for high amine foods like chocolate and cheese. Dietary sources of toxic amines are meat, dairy, chocolate, avocados, raisins, and fermented foods. Stress, infection, and pathogens also create toxic amines, and raise MAO levels.

I hope I haven't gotten too complicated here with all this talk of amines, and MAO. Don't worry if you have to read all this stuff ten times over to get it. All you really need to understand is that when you eat chocolate the reactions that follow will eventually lead to lower levels of serotonin in the brain and that stimulates cravings for more chocolate, and other carbohydrates.

STOP CHOCOLATE CRAVINGS

STEP ONE
Low serotonin is the most common cause of chocolate cravings, so treat it as instructed under Carbohydrate Cravings.

STEP TWO
Low blood sugar is the next most common cause. Treat as instructed under Sugar Cravings.

STEP THREE
Take a magnesium supplement. The safest way to take magnesium is as a calcium-magnesium combination supplement.

STEP FOUR
Eliminate fat cravings.

STEP FIVE
Check adrenal function in Salt Craving section.

STEP SIX
Stimulate your endorphins. There are lots of techniques to stimulate endorphins. Try one of these:

1. Smell something you find pleasant. Flowers work well for most people. Essential oils are also a convienient source of pleasant smells. Find one that appeals to you and keep it around to sniff whenever you need the boost. My favorites

are ylang ylang, peppermint, spearmint, wintergreen, fir, beech and cinnamon.

2. Exercise will produce endorphins. The more vigorous better. Athletes are experts at utilizing this effect. If you're out of shape it won't be very effective until you get in better condition.

3. Sunshine

4. Sweet tasting foods can trick your brain into releasing endorphins. To get this effect without sugar try glycine, stevia, or cinnamon. For more ideas see my book "Sweet Solutions" (also available from Bio-Science, see *Sources*). It gives lots of healthy alternatives to aspartame, sugar, honey and high carbohydrate sweeteners

5. Sing

6. Take a hot bath

7. Meditate

8. For more ideas see *The Sweetest Food of All—Endorphins*

CHAPTER 8

PROTEIN CRAVINGS

Protein craving can result from protein deficiency. Just eating protein is not enough. You must digest it. A deficiency of stomach acid or digestive enzymes could result in improper digestion. Poor digestion of protein can lead to bad breath, gas, constipation, and other problems. To test for stomach acid production, see instructions under Sour Cravings. Even if this test shows ample stomach acid you may still need digestive enzymes. Extensive metabolic tests on urine can be used to indicate your ability to digest protein.

When protein is craved there may be problems with parasites. The parasites can be as small as one cell or up to several feet long. They can be lodged in the intestines, or migrate anywhere in the body. Of the thousands of potential parasites found worldwide most healthy people have at least a few. It is rare (but not impossible) to find someone 100% free of any parasites.

Parasites have numerous methods of creating food cravings to keep you feeding them. Their favorite foods are fats, sugars and proteins. One type of tapeworm absorbs Vitamin B12. You gradually become deficient in this important vitamin. One of the best food sources of Vitamin B12 is meat. You crave meat to replenish your B12, but alas it is all in vain. Any B12 you do eat is quickly absorbed by the worm. Other parasites may induce B12 deficiency by simply inhibiting your ability to absorb it. Eventually, you become anemic from B12 deficiency, but only after years of deficiency, long after the parasite has completed its life cycle.

Parasites also generate ammonia and other waste products. Ammonia is toxic, especially to the brain. These toxins add to the burden that the kidneys, and liver must eliminate. They deplete the liver of amino acids like glycine, and glutamate that are used up in the removal of this toxic waste.

Vitamin and mineral deficiencies can also lead to meat cravings. Meat is an excellent source of many vitamins and minerals, including: B12, iron and copper.

The solutions to protein cravings can be as simple as taking a parasite medication, or as complex as determining total vitamin, mineral, and nutritional status. Protein cravings may indicate a serious deficiency or disease that needs to be addressed.

TO STOP PROTEIN CRAVINGS

STEP ONE
Test for adequate stomach acid. See "Sour Cravings" section on this procedure. You may need to do this before the craving actually strikes. If uncertain you can skip to Step Two until this testing can be completed. One way to replace deficient stomach acid is to take a product like **"Betaine HCL"** or **"HCL PLUS"** *(see Sources)*. A visit to your local health food store will uncover even more brands. One tablet is usually adequate if the meal is small. See the Sour Section for further suggestions.

Taking excessive dietary acids, even to replace missing stomach acid can lead to excessive acid build-up in the body. It must be balanced by acid neutralizing foods, primarily fresh vegetables, and sometimes timely consumption of basic solutions like Alka Seltzer in the evening (and when the stomach is empty). Getting the stomach back to normal acid production is the ultimate goal.

STEP TWO

Eat a small amount of **protein** with lots of digestive enzymes. Try 4 oz. high protein food with 6 **digestive enzyme** capsules. Be sure the enzymes have protease included. I like "**Multizyme**" (see *Sources*).

STEP THREE

1. Take a balanced **multiple vitamin-mineral** supplement.
2. Take 6 each of : **1000 mcg B12 and 400 mcg folic acid** lozenges, chew slowly. If your lozenges are of a different strength, adjust the amount.

STEP FOUR

Take an amino acid supplement. Be sure it includes extra:

    l-Glycine   l-Cysteine   l-Arginine

STEP FIVE

Identify and eliminate **parasites.** You may need expert help to accomplish this.

STEP SIX

Test for fat cravings, these are often the true source of a craving for a food that's high in fat and protein.

CHAPTER 9

SOUR FOODS

PICKLES, SAUERKRAUT & VINEGAR

Sour food cravings can indicate chemical imbalances requiring a neutralization of excess acids. It begins with overconsumption of acid forming foods. These are sugars, carbohydrates, grains, meats, and most cooked foods. Overexertion, fatigue, acute infections and poor metabolism can also lead to acid accumulations. Your system eventually becomes too acidic. Now you begin to crave acids. This occurs because many tart tasting foods will actually result in a net loss of acid after digestion. The common use of fresh lemon juice to restore balance, works by reducing acids in your system. Unfortunately vinegar and other refined and processed acids increase the acid in your system. The long term solution is to increase consumption of fresh fruits and vegetables, and cut back on the acid forming foods. It is also possible, but rare, to crave sour foods due to an over alkaline condition. It can be a problem with some vegetarians that eat lots of vegetables and fruits. With sour cravings you must first determine if the problem is due to acid, alkaline imbalance, or stomach problems.

To determine the difference you'll need some pH test paper. I like the rolls of thin tape. Collect a urine sample and use a strip of the test paper to measure pH. The paper will turn color immediately, telling you the pH of your urine. Less than 7 is acid, over 7 is alkaline, and 7 is neutral. Drink as much water as you can during this procedure to assist your system in rebalancing its chemistry. Keep in mind the urine naturally changes pH throughout the day, and this test is for determining your present condition only.

FOR ACID URINE
Immediately take 2 **Alka-Seltzer Gold** tablets or a teaspoon of baking soda dissolved in a glass of water. Wait 15 minutes and re-test your urine if you still crave sours. Repeat as needed.

FOR ALKALINE URINE
Drink a tablespoon of **apple cider vinegar** in a glass of water to reverse alkaline conditions. Wait 15 minutes and re-test your urine if the craving still exists. Use only natural apple cider vinegar, (preferably raw). Repeat as needed. Yoga, and chiropractic adjustments can often help people with excessive alkaline conditions. Chronic disease can also be a cause of alkaline conditions.

STOMACH TROUBLES
Abdominal distress from overeating fatty foods can sometimes lead to an acid craving. This may also occur when the stomach is not producing enough stomach acid and instinctively we

seek some acid to assist digestion. You can easily test yourself to determine if you are producing enough stomach acid.

TEST FOR STOMACH ACID
Breakfast and Lunch: Eat small low fat meals.

Test meal: Around 4pm eat a can of beets, juice and all.
Dinner: Eat a small meal of low fat foods after 7pm, if desired. You can skip dinner if the beets were enough to satisfy.

RESULTS
Collect a urine sample. Normal urine is pale yellow. The natural red compounds in beets require acid to break them down. If you have adequate stomach acid production, your sample will be yellow. If the urine is pink it indicates low stomach acid. The darker red it is the more severe the problem. Any result that indicates low stomach acid needs to be further tested. Digestive enzymes, and other digestive aids may be indicated. If you don't like or can't eat beets, there are vegetable dyes that you can take as a pill to test stomach acid, (see sources).

If you test low on stomach acid you should supplement meals with at least:

Glutamic Acid HCL (50 mg)
Taurine (1000 mg)
Histamine (2000 mg)
Salt (1/2 teaspoon)
B6 (100mg)

These supplements aid your stomach in production of stomach acid.

In addition you can temporarily add 150 mg of Betaine HCL (Caution this may eventually lead to excess acids).

If you test high in stomach acid and you know that you have digestive troubles due to irritated stomach or intestines, such as colitis, ulcer, or diverticulitis, you can try the "cabbage cure." Sip **fresh raw cabbage juice**, about a quart daily. You'll need to invest in a juicer, and buy cabbage in bulk but this cure has worked for thousands. It usually takes 6–8 weeks to heal the irritation. If you want a more convenient solution, the active ingredient has been isolated from cabbage and is available in pill form as **gastrazyme.**

You must also consider salt craving when the sour food craved also contains salt, such as pickles and sauerkraut.

CHAPTER 10

SPICY FOODS

Pepper, cayenne, chili, ginger, mustard, cloves, onions, garlic, and horseradish are all hot foods. They contain substances that have been identified to induce a variety of physical effects. When a child or adult first tastes these foods there is an immediate repulsion. Similarly, animals also show aversion to these foods. Animals can not be conditioned or trained to eat hot spicy foods. People on the other hand often report a craving for one or more of these foods. There are several possible explanations for this difference.

The reaction to eating spicy foods includes increased saliva, flushing and sweating on the face and chest, nasal secretions, and tearing. All these reflexes aid the removal of the noxious substance. This initial painful reaction with the subsequent reflexes results in a stimulation of the mucus membranes, a flush or rush of adrenaline, a stimulation of the entire digestive tract, improved circulation, improved blood fat profiles (shown for at least some of these foods), death of bacteria and possibly other types of pathogens. All of these side effects are medicinal. They are usually beneficial. Cayenne in particular has also been shown to affect pain receptors. The cayenne depletes the pain nerves of substance P, needed to stimulate the nerves. Once the initial pain subsides further pain is inhibited.

This feature has enabled cayenne to be used effectively in pain control with arthritis and other chronic pain. Tabasco sauce has been shown to kill bacteria in food, and thereby reduce the risk of food-borne illness. Onions and garlic have long been known for their medicinal value in a number of conditions. Ginger is a popular remedy for stomach ache, colds, and motion sickness.

Besides the medicinal value of spicy foods, they have one other unusual feature. They make bitter foods taste a little bit less bitter. This is probably not the reason why spicy foods are craved, but may help explain why beer drinkers often like spicy foods. The spicy foods makes the beer less bitter tasting. We know that animals will crave bizarre foods when ill, but will they eat spicy foods when ill? The research remains to be done in this field. Why do people crave spicy foods? The answer may relate to the side effects.

The most obvious effect is on digestion. If you crave spicy food you may have digestive troubles. Perhaps they are minor, and the stimulation from the spicy foods provides the needed effect. If you feel your digestion is fine and still you crave spicy foods, the craving may be masking some minor digestive problem with the medicinal effect of the spicy food. Anyone eating the typical western diet of mostly cooked foods, some fried foods, and lots of refined sugar and flour, is stressing their digestive system, even if they don't realize it yet.

The adrenals are small glands located just above each kidney.

They produce adrenaline in times of stress. This adrenaline stimulates the entire body and mind. It wakes you up and gets everything into high gear. Constant stress, nutritional deficiencies, or toxins can weaken the adrenals. Once depleted they may not function as intended. You can test your adrenal function with the tests in Salt Cravings. This will indicate possible adrenal malfunction. Spicy foods stimulate the adrenals, giving you that "adrenaline rush". Your metabolism is also temporarily increased by this stimulation. Craving spicy foods may indicate a need for stimulation due to weak adrenals.

To summarize spicy food cravings can be the result of an instinctive desire for:
1. chronic pain relief (primarily abdominal)
2. relief from congested sinuses
3. digestive problems
4. enhanced taste—ability to tolerate bitter foods
5. adrenal stimulation
6. killing of pathogens in food
7. increased metabolism

Because all of the known effects from spicy foods are beneficial, this is one craving you should indulge in moderation. Naturally if the spicy food is also high in salt or fat or something else that is not beneficial you should test and eliminate those cravings. People with ulcers or other digestive irritations may wonder if these hot foods will irritate their ulcers. While it may feel like these foods burn, only a few like the hot Jalapeño peppers, actually irritate. Most spicy foods just give the sensation of burning. If in doubt about your particular condition be sure to ask your doctor.

Craving spicy foods should alert you to the possible cause. Now is the time to find out what is wrong with you and fix it. Giving in to these cravings is OK for now, and possibly the best thing you can do for the moment. Discovering the cause and eliminating it will still allow you the pleasure of indulging in spicy foods. It is only the actual craving of food that we are trying to eliminate, not the pleasure of eating. Once the craving is gone you may be pleasantly surprised to find you actually enjoy the food more but are now in full control of when and how much you care to eat. Recognizing the underlying cause and treating it before it becomes a bigger problem will improve your health while eliminating these cravings.

CHAPTER 11

COFFEE, CAFFEINE & SOFT DRINKS

CAFFEINE

Caffeine is found in chocolate, headache medicines, coffee, teas, and most soda pop. It is stimulating and generally beneficial in small amounts. The problem occurs when levels become excessive. Because it is hidden in soda pop, candy and medicines, it's easy to overindulge. Excessive caffeine can lead to irritability and sleeplessness. Excessive caffeine can aggravate food cravings by disrupting the blood sugar levels. Caffeine is addictive and because we develop a tolerance to caffeine it is easy to gradually keep increasing the amount until suddenly you realize that you're hooked. Stopping cold turkey is difficult. Headaches can be triggered during withdrawal. Slowly decreasing your caffeine each day is the safest way to break the cycle. Homeopathic remedies have also been useful to many people in eliminating withdrawal side effects. Anything over 5 cups of coffee or tea is probably excessive. The amount of caffeine in sodas, chocolate and medicines should also be considered.

COFFEE

Coffee has more than just caffeine to consider. It also contains benzoic acid. The benzoic acid is mildly toxic. To remove the benzoic acid, your liver combines it with the amino acid glycine to form hippuric acid. Hippuric acid is easily excreted by the kidneys. While moderate amounts of these acids alone won't cause a glycine shortage, big coffee drinkers may need to supplement their diet with extra glycine. Because glycine is one of the most abundant amino acids in our body an abundant supply is essential. Fortunately we are able to manufacture glycine. Additional dietary glycine can also enhance health when the demand is heavy. Besides the vital role glycine plays in detoxifying and removing poisons, it is essential in making strong connective tissue. Fingernail condition is one easy way to judge the strength of your connective tissue. Strong fingernails need ample glycine to form. Some women eat gelatin to help improve their fingernails. The high glycine content of gelatin explains how gelatin can help to form strong fingernails.

SOFT DRINKS

I consider healthy food and drink to be those items that you can consume in relatively large portions on a regular basis without suffering any ill effects, and hopefully providing you with some if not all the essential nutrients required for healthy bodies. Pure water can fit most of this description but the only nutrient it usually supplies is H2O. Relatively large portions are the amounts that average people consume in the course of their day. Even water can be consumed to excess. Most food and drink contains some toxins that our body must eliminate. When the amount of most toxins is small, or the amount consumed is small, a healthy liver and kidneys can easily

eliminate them. Not all
toxins are so easy to get rid
of. Certain heavy metals
and fat soluble toxins
may lodge in the brain
and tissues, making re-
moval more difficult.
Some health professionals
have questioned the extensive use of aluminum in food

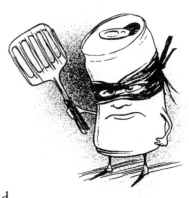

packaging (soda cans) and cooking utensils. Aluminum can be
a toxic metal and it accumulates in brain tissues. The acids in
certain foods including soda pop may assist the aluminum to
dissolve into the beverage. While the amount in solution is
minute the effects of metal toxicity are cumulative and poorly
understood by current medical researchers. The old fashioned
glass bottles did not have this problem.

Cravings for soft drinks may be due to the caffeine, sugars,
aspartame, acids, or carbonation. The caffeine found in many
of these drinks may actually be the least of your worries.
Children are more sensitive to the effects of caffeine so their
risk of overdose is greater. The sugar in the form of high
fructose corn syrup or aspartame that is used to sweeten soda
pop worries me the most.

Aspartame, also known as Nutra-Sweet or Equal, has been
linked to brain tumors, and a host of neurological diseases,
according to H.J.Roberts, M.D., author of *Aspartame
(NutraSweet™): Is It Safe?* Many other health professionals
also share his concern.

Sugars, including high fructose corn syrup also have problems.

They can create an initial high blood sugar level, with a low blood sugar rebound. The type of sugar used to make soda pop is usually high fructose corn syrup because it's very inexpensive. Your liver must then convert this fructose into glucose so that you can use it. The effort required by the liver to convert fructose has been compared to the effort your liver must make in detoxifying alcoholic beverages. While you won't get drunk on fructose, your liver will be taxed if you consume large amounts. See *Sugar Cravings* to control these urges. Essential trace minerals and vitamins may also be depleted when excess fructose is consumed.

Animal studies with rats showed that fructose seems to interfere with copper metabolism. Rats fed a diet with some copper deficiency showed typical signs of copper deficiency, but when fructose replaced sucrose in those copper deficient diets, the heart, liver, testes, and pancreas were damaged, eventually leading to death. Copper is essential to many enzymes and deficiencies in copper may be related to many diseases. The copper jewelry that some arthritic patients find of benefit may be due to the small amount of copper that is absorbed through the skin.

Carbonation in soft drinks increases the permeability of the blood-brain barrier. This allows all the chemicals in soda pop to reach higher concentrations in the brain. The blood-brain barrier exists to protect us from potentially toxic chemicals. The carbonation of soft drinks allows these chemicals easy access to our brain. If you are craving soft drinks you may be craving the way this carbonation enhances the chemical changes resulting from the sugars, aspartame, or caffeine. You may also be craving the way these acids and carbonation change your pH (See *Sour Foods* to evaluate your pH).

STOPPING THESE CRAVINGS

If you replace the item craved with a healthy beverage, you can still get the endorphins and stimulation without the problems. Fortunately there are great substitutes for coffee, tea, and sodas. All hot drinks, even hot water will stimulate your body and aid digestion. Postum, Pero and several other products are excellent coffee substitutes. Herbal teas can also be a healthy substitute. Soda can be replaced with vitamin C beverages that use carbonated vitamin C products, such as Bio-C or C-Salts to give fizz to flavored drinks. To make these I take about 1 cup fruit, 1 cup water, 1 tsp glycine and 1 tsp glycerine to taste for sweetness and 1 tsp Bio-C, blend to make a refreshing beverage. Seltzer water can also be flavored as a substitute.

Additional steps to control low blood sugar and low serotonin will probably be necessary and are listed under carbohydrate cravings.

CHAPTER 12

ALCOHOL

WINE, BEER & ADULT BEVERAGES

Bright lights alone can reduce the craving for alcohol by 90%. Doctors in Vienna, Austria treated alcoholics from 6am to 10:30pm with room lighting three times brighter than normal. This resulted in 1/10th the medication needed, and better moods for the patients. If possible, outside exposure to the sun would be ideal. If inside lighting is necessary, buy some extra lights—as many as you can afford and keep them on all day. The most effective colors are blue and violet, but white will work just fine.

Melatonin is produced in a cyclic manner according to light and dark exposure. The effect of bright lights may only work when total darkness follows, allowing for melatonin production. **Melatonin** has been shown to decrease the craving for alcohol and should be considered in treating this problem. Read the Melatonin Section to see if this is for you.

Alcohol cravings often respond to the treatment for **low blood sugar.** Try the steps under *Carbohydrate Cravings—Sweets*, to treat the low blood sugar problem.

All alcoholics have **nutritional deficiencies.** Eliminating the deficiencies can go a long way in controlling the cravings. Virtually every nutrient needs to be supplemented, especially the anti-oxidant nutrients. The anti-oxidants and liver specific nutrients include but are not limited to: **Lipoic acid, vitamin A, all the B vitamins (especially B6), vitamin C, vitamin D, vitamin E, Omega-3 oils (flax and fish oils), selenium, bioflavonoids, milk thistle extracts, l-cysteine, and l-methionine.**

Herbs commonly used to help stop alcohol cravings are:
Kudzu
Cayenne
Golden Seal
Passion Flower
Saw Palmetto
Skullcap
Valerian

CHAPTER 13

TOBACCO

CIGARETTES, CIGARS, PIPES AND CHEW

I don't want to argue the merits or faults of tobacco. It has proven health risks, as well as some potential benefits. The issue here is how to stop the craving for tobacco. First as with any other habit, you must want to stop. If you enjoy tobacco, and don't really want to quit, then you probably won't. If you honestly want to stop, then try the following methods, they really do help reduce the craving. But nothing will make you stop. First you must want to stop.

Several herbs have been identified that actually reduce the physical craving. I recommend giving them all a try.

HERBS AND SUPPLEMENT

AVENA SATIVA

Commonly called oats. It is the alkaloid avenine contained in oats that stimulates the nervous system, and has been used in India to treat opium addicts. It has been shown to reduce the amount of cigarettes smoked in research studies. (Nature 71;229:496) Large doses of this extract can cause headaches, so be cautious when using the extract. Oats can be eaten daily, but will be much, much weaker in effect than the prepared extract.

LOBELIA INFLATA

Commonly called Indian tobacco, asthma weed and pukeweed among other names. It also contains an alkaloid lobeline, which has properties similar to nicotine. It is included in many anti-smoking products in Europe. Overdoses of lobelia can induce nausea and vomiting, so be careful with this herb.

CALAMUS ROOT

In high doses it can induce nausea and vomiting, but it is considered one of the most effective in curbing the appetite for smoking. It also aids in liquefying mucus to clear congestion.

VITAMIN C

Try taking 1000–5000 mg daily of vitamin C. Use the buffered, or pH neutral type. Several studies have shown vitamin C to assist in reducing the desire to smoke. This a relatively safe vitamin and some people have used even higher amounts. The dose works best if taken gradually throughout the day.

TRYPTOPHAN

Tryptophan decreases tobacco cravings. See Carbohydrate Cravings for steps to increase tryptophan levels.

ZINC

Cadmium is a toxic metal found in smoke. It displaces zinc, leaving many smokers with zinc deficiency.

STOMACH PROBLEMS

Smokers are prone to low stomach acid. You can test this using the instructions in the *Sour Foods* section.

ANXIETY OR APATHY

See the first chapter for stress and anxiety formulas, especially "**Calma**". If you want to make up your own blend be sure to use:

l-Histidine	GABA
l-Glycine	l-Taurine
l-Tryptophan (Spirulina is the best food source)	
B1	B2
B6	Vitamin C
Calcium	Magnesium
Zinc	

The stimulation from nicotine can help to get you going in the morning. A natural alternative to nicotine are these amino acids. They stimulate best if taken first thing in the morning on an empty stomach. The usual dosage is 1-2 grams. If you have high blood pressure these may aggravate it further, so consult your doctor if necessary and start with a much lower dose.

l-Phenylalanine	l-Tyrosine
l-Methionine	

Read about other options in the sections on:
Compulsive Eating
Carbohydrate Cravings

The Sweetest Food of All—Endorphins
Homeopathy
Acupuncture
Breaking Habits

I *do not* recommend these two tricks, as they rarely work:

1. Nicotine-containing gums or patches. These may make the initial break easier but ultimately the gum or patch must be stopped. Many users resume smoking.

2. Hypnosis: this helps some people but many eventually resume smoking again.

CHAPTER 14

DRUGS

COCAINE AND OTHER PRESCRIPTIONS

The craving for drugs is similar to the craving for foods. Cocaine has been shown to block the uptake of serotonin. The result is an increased craving due to low serotonin, the same problem faced in Carbohydrate Cravings. While whole books could be written on curing drug habits including prescription and illegal drugs, I won't attempt anything that monumental here. I would like to point out that the methods presented throughout this book to reduce food cravings have also been shown to reduce drug cravings. While several treatment centers have implemented these therapies, they still remain vastly under-utilized.

As with food cravings, these techniques will not create a distaste for the substance, they will simply reduce the craving. The desire to stop using the drug must exist first. Then these methods can be useful tools.

Start using the techniques for carbohydrate cravings that increase serotonin levels. Treat other cravings as they occur and be sure to use ample endorphin stimulators.

CHAPTER 15

MELATONIN

Melatonin is a hormone with many functions. Many people know of its popular use in inducing sleep, and resetting your diurnal clock. It also improves health by protecting cells from damaging free radicals. Melatonin is important in regulating our cycles of sleep and activity. In minute amounts, it affects our moods and brain chemistry. Maximum health and maximum melatonin production occurs around age 20, and almost every disease studied shows excessively low melatonin including depression, alcoholism, schizophrenia, chronic pain, cancer, arthritis, AIDS, hearts disease, Alzheimer's, PMS and cataracts.

We know that melatonin decreases with aging, and levels of melatonin are very low with most diseases. Melatonin can be further lowered by aspirin, ibuprofen, sleeping pills, caffeine found in chocolate, coffee, tea and most soda pop, tobacco, alcohol, electromagnetic fields produced by electrical appliances or high power lines, and many prescription drugs. This includes most heart medications and high blood pressure medications, steroids, antidepressants, and anti-anxiety drugs, and even vitamin B12 if given in massive doses.

Can melatonin stop food cravings? There have been studies to indicate it does help, especially in sweet, starch and alcohol cravings. The evidence suggests it may help other cravings as well since it normalizes brain chemistry in some very significant ways. This is a new field and I'm sure as new research reveals more about this hormone, the recommendations could change. If you want to incorporate melatonin in your quest for health, here are some basic guide lines.

Melatonin should never be given to children, it delays puberty, and may have other ill effects.

Melatonin should be avoided by: people on steroid drugs, pregnant or nursing mothers, women during ovulation as it may suppress ovulation, people with severe allergic or autoimmune diseases unless under doctor's supervision.

Melatonin should probably not be taken during the day. This is in direct opposition to the natural cycle. Some studies suggest taking melatonin during the day may stimulate cancer cells and exacerbate mental illness. Nighttime use is the only time melatonin is considered safe and useful. Therapeutic dosages of .1 mg to 75 mg are used for a variety of conditions. However, common dosages ranges between 1–10 mg taken at bedtime.

Melatonin works well for 90% of the people, but 10% report side effects. The most common are increased alertness, with resulting insomnia, and headaches. These "reactors" usually have other health problems, but the reason why they react adversely is still a mystery. Some people react at certain times and mysteriously don't at other times. One possible problem could be an allergic reaction to the filler used to make the tablet or capsule. Another brand may work if this is the problem. Uncovering the problem requires the assistance of a health professional.

CHAPTER 16

ENDORPHINS

THE SWEETEST FOOD OF ALL

Endorphins are those brain chemicals that relieve pain. More importantly they produce the sensations of pleasure. They are the ultimate goal in most cravings. Love and affection are the source of our strongest pleasures and also our strongest cravings. While food can be a substitute for love, it only temporarily satisfies us. Happiness and love with their ultimate results also give the ultimate "high." The survival benefit is obvious and vital for procreation. Ultimately happiness comes from within, after the cravings have been controlled.

A spouse or close friend is only one way to share and thereby increase joy and happiness. Sometimes your best friend is a beloved pet. Pets can be especially loving, with boundless and unconditional affection that often appears to be their sole purpose in life.

Food cravings can interfere with our mental functions. They can influence emotional cravings and behavior. Can you really be happy when you crave chocolate? How can you fully love anyone, yourself especially, when all you think about is food? By eliminating the food cravings, you can improve normal mental functions. Now the mind can become free to love fully.

Endorphins are the key to happiness and joy. Don't wait around. Make some for yourself! You can never have enough. Eating does stimulate endorphins but there are also calorie free options like:

1. Laughing

2. Smiling

3. A massage—getting one

4. Smelling something pleasant—flowers work well

5. Singing

6. Meditating

7. Taking a hot bath

8. Spending quality time with a loved one

9. Exercising

10. Getting out in the sunshine

11. Using the techniques in acupressure to stimulate endorphins

12. Fooling your tongue with something sweet that's healthy such as cinnamon, vanilla, nutmeg or stevia

13. There is a joy that comes from the satisfaction of a task well done. Try completing some small task every day

CHAPTER 17

HOMEOPATHY

I struggled for a long time in deciding if I should add this chapter. Many prominent scientists and doctors believe that homeopathy is worthless and the only effect it may have is that of a placebo. I also once shared their belief so I can understand their position. It is not my intent to try and convince others of the validity of homeopathy. Just a few short years ago acupuncture was also accused of being a worthless placebo. Acupuncture is now recognized as a valid treatment and useful anaesthetic for surgery. Perhaps homeopathy will soon begin to get the recognition it deserves.

Homeopathy is the use of activated carrier substances to trigger some sort of physical change. Water and lactose are commonly used as carriers. By careful and precise percussing of the carrier with various substances a homeopathic dilution is formed. Those who firmly believe that these dilute carriers can not have any effect base their opinion on the fact that current accepted scientific theory cannot explain the mechanism. Other scientists in an effort to prove the validity or nonsense of homeopathy have done extensive testing. Much to their surprise the results indicate homeopathy has a measurable and testable effect. This effect can not be explained by current scientific beliefs.

I am not going to offer any explanation as to how or why homeopathy works. I can not prove my personal theory. The effect is not a placebo effect that much has been proven. Before medicine knew about infectious agents like bacteria, it was accepted knowledge that evil spirits caused disease. One observant doctor noticed that if he washed his hands between patients he could stop or severely limit the spread of childbirth fever. He tried in vain to get other doctors to wash also, but they refused. After all, how could washing hands have anything to do with evil spirits. The point is that I don't need to understand how homeopathy works to be able to benefit from it. Someday science will give us the answer. Until then if it's safe, effective, and low cost, I will continue to use it until something better comes along.

Many people have cured their food cravings and other health problems using only homeopathy. Unfortunately it doesn't work for everyone. The reason may be in the application. Homeopathy is currently more of an art than a science. There are thousands of remedies, available in dozens of potencies. Finding the correct dose and the correct remedy can be a complex puzzle. The study and application of homeopathic remedies can take many years to master. It is also possible to have beginners luck, and some doctors seem to have a certain instinct or intuition at finding the correct remedy. Homeopathic doctors are common in Europe and gaining popularity in the United States. The best way to find a good homeopath is by word of mouth. Ask around to find someone that is getting good results.

If you want to study up on the remedies and learn more about this field there are lots of good books. The following chart shows some of the commonly available homeopathic remedies that have been found to be useful for treating cravings. No list of possible remedies is ever complete. The following is only a starting place, using commonly available remedies. I have tried to limit the possible remedies to those that have been found most useful. There are hundreds more possible remedies. The ideal remedy for each person takes into account many more physical and emotional symptoms than just the cravings. If you are attempting to treat yourself you should research the potential remedy before treatment to determine if you fit most of the typical symptoms for that remedy.

I hesitate to mention this next option. It is possible to make your own homeopathic remedy. The preparation is not difficult but the slightest sloppiness of even one step will render the final product worthless. Read all the instructions several times before attempting this and don't be fooled into thinking it's easy because it is not. Because it is virtually cost free to everyone, this option appeals to all those thrifty people that have the inclination to be self-sufficient. Start with a small sample of the item you crave, for example salt. You'll need 50 small grains of salt, or about one very small pinch. Use a clean spoon to handle the salt, put it into a small clean glass jar or vial. The glass jar must be absolutely clean. Only use a brand new jar, and even then rinse it and the cap out at least ten times with distilled water to get any traces of dust out. To the jar and salt, add about 10cc distilled water and cap. There should be ample air space above the liquid level. Now you are going to shake the jar very vigorously. This step is called "percussing" and is crucial. One hundred and fifty shakes are required. The exact force required in each shake is also important. Too much or too little and the product will be inferior. Without personal supervision it is difficult to explain how to properly shake but I will attempt it anyway. First, prepare a surface onto which you can strike the jar. One historical favorite was a large book with a leather cover. The book's surface was firm enough to absorb some of the impact, while the cover provided enough protection to avoid breaking the jar. Try to duplicate this surface by using a hard surface like a counter or large book covered with a thin but firm padding like leather. You will also need to take into account the jar or vial you will be using as to how much concussion it can tolerate. To provide the force, hold the jar in your hand about 8–10 inches above your prepared surface, and rest your elbow comfortably on or near the surface. Bring the jar into contact with the surface by allowing your hand to fall towards the surface. The surface will absorb the impact. Only the jar should make contact with the surface. *Caution*: Do not break the jar! Wear protective gloves and glasses when first trying this so that if the glass does break you won't get hurt. Practice is essential to get a comfortable but effective stroke. Continue for the full 150 beats. Once prepared this solution is called your first extraction. Some items may form better extracts if you use alcohol such as vodka instead of water for this first extraction. Now carefully take 1cc of this extraction and place it into a new clean jar adding another 10cc distilled water and then percussing again for 150 stokes. Continue this dilution and percussing process for 6 or more times. Each solution you have made is a homeopathic solution of differing strength.

The actual strength that will work best for you is impossible to predict. You will need to simply try different strengths to see if they work. As a general rule the more dilute solutions work better at resolving chronic and long-standing problems. To use simply take a few drops, say 10–20, and place them in your mouth. Hold for as long as possible before swallowing. You must not have eaten or drunk anything in the last 30 minutes before using.

Another vital consideration in preparing homeopathic remedies is the fact that any contamination—even the touch of your finger on the inside of the cap can ruin the batch. Strong odors, perfumes, magnetic or electrical fields can also ruin the batch. Climate or seasonal changes may also affect the batch, as can the phase of the moon. In short, home-made homeopathic remedies are variable in their quality. They must also be used immediately or re-shaken before use if allowed to sit for even one day. Drops must be taken out in such a way that the rest of the jar is not contaminated by an eyedropper or spoon. Because of all these problems, I usually use commercially prepared remedies. They have been manufactured under strict conditions, and when prepared in pill form are easy to dispense without contamination of the batch. The pill form is more stable and can sit on a shelf for months or perhaps longer and still be effective. All homeopathics should be kept away from sunlight, and strong odors.

The following table lists some commercially available remedies and common cravings associated with their use.

FOOD CRAVED	REMEDIES
Alcoholic Drinks	Arsenicum Album Capsicum Crotalus Horridus Lachesis Nux Vomica Sulphur Selenium
Beer	Aconitum Napellus Nux Vomica Sulphur
Brandy	Nux Vomica Opium
Whiskey	Lac Caninum Sulphur
Wine	Phosphorus Sulphur China officinalis
Bread	Mercurius Vivus
Chocolate	Lepidium Bonariense Lyssin (Hydrophobium)
Coffee	Angustura Vera

FOOD CRAVED	REMEDIES
Cold Drinks	Aconitum Napellus Arenicum Album Bryonia Alba Chamomilla China Officinalis Cina Eupatorium Perfoliatum Mercurius Vivus Mercurius Corrosivus Natrum Sulphuricum Phosphorus Veratrinum Album
Cold Food	Phosphorus Pulsatilla Nigricans
Fat	Nitricum Acidum Mezereum Arsenicum Album
Acid Fruit	Phosphoricum Acidum Veratrinum Album
Herring	Nitricum Acidum
Spicy Food	China Officinalis Phosphorus Sulphur
Ice	Veratrinum Album

FOOD CRAVED	REMEDIES
Ice Cream	Phosphorus
Dirt, Chalk, Dlay, Pencils	Nitricum Acidum Cina
Meat	Ferrum Metallicum Natrum Muriaticum
Smoked foods	Causticum Tuberculinum Tarentula Hispanica
Milk	Rhus Toxicodendron
Oysters	Lachesis
Salty Foods	Argentum Nitricum Carbo Vegetabilis Lac Caninum Natrum Muriaticum Phosphorus Veratrinum Album
Sour Foods	Corallium Rubrum Hepar Sulphuris Calcareum Veratrinum Album
Sweets	Argentum Nitricum China Officinalis Lycopodium Sulphur Argentum Nitricum

FOOD CRAVED	REMEDIES
Tobacco	Tabacum Staphisagria Nux Vomica Lobelia Inflata
Vinegar	Hepar Sulphuric Calcareum

Strange things during Pregnancy: Lyssin (Hydrophobinum)

For Irritable moods try Staphisagria

CHAPTER 18

ACUPRESSURE

Acupuncture is the practice of inserting needles into trigger points to restore health or to stop pain. Acupressure is a simpler, safer and self-administered method to achieve similar effects. Both methods have been used for centuries to stop food cravings and other addictions. Like homeopathy, full understanding of the mechanism remains to be discovered. We do know that it can be a powerful stimulator of brain endorphins. This would explain one mechanism that stops cravings. These methods can be the key to lasting success in treating addictions of all types.

Locating trigger points that need stimulation can be easy if you know where to look. Any sore spot on the body is potentially a treatment point. Naturally, injured locations will be sore, but injuries should never be stimulated, only healthy tissue. The pressure varies with the location but should always be gentle, and brief. Never press harder than five pounds pressure, and one pound or less in delicate areas, like the head. Slow circular motions works best. Treat for 10 to 20 seconds only. Longer times may lead to bruising, something that you want to avoid. You can repeat the treatment three times or more daily until the area is no longer sore when tested. You can often get even better results using light, magnets or electricity to stimulate the points. Several battery operated electrical devices have been used extensively in Russia and are now available in the United States. Light in the 650 to 690 wavelength range has been used both as lasers and diodes to stimulate these points. These devices are now affordable to most people for personal use and are priced around $150 or less. Magnets can also stimulate these points. When using magnets, ALWAYS use the positive pole. This is the same charge as the North Pole of the earth. Mixed or negative poles can have irritating effects or worse. There are certain conditions that respond better to South Pole magnets, but the risk of using them outweighs the benefits in almost every case. It is far safer to stick with safe and effective North Pole energies.

The following diagrams illustrate areas you need to explore for tenderness. Any tender spot becomes a treatment point.

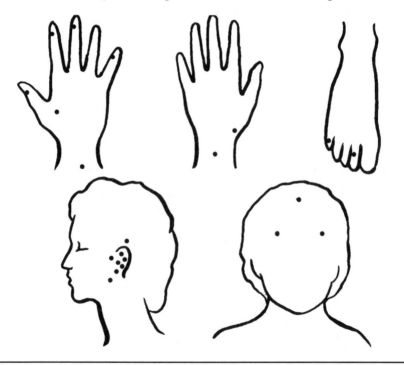

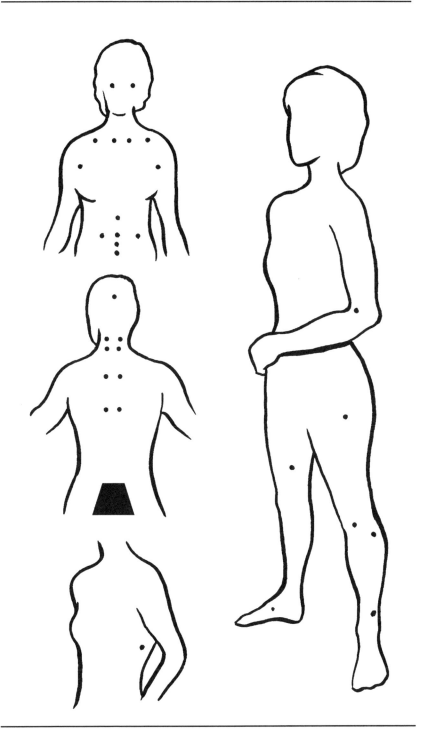

CHAPTER 19

BREAKING HABITS

SMELLS OR THOUGHTS TRIGGERING CRAVINGS

After hunger, the most powerful stimulus to eating, is probably the odor of a favorite food. The smell of popcorn, caramel corn, pizza, baking bread, barbecued ribs, coffee, or almost anything you crave can be overpowering. Even if you have recently eaten, the odor makes you eat again. You don't actually even need the smell, just the thought can be enough. Did reading the above reference to several foods tempt you. Do you crave chocolate every time you think about your grandmother, who always gave you a chocolate bar when you visited? Our brains are very good at making associations between food and odors, or food and behaviors. To survive and adapt, primitive brains learned quickly what odors meant food. The odor also conditioned us to anticipate and prepare for the food. The digestive system is turned on and insulin is released to prepare for incoming food. These reactions ultimately increase cravings by altering blood sugar and brain chemicals.

Now that you know it is just a trained association between the smell or idea of the food and the actual craving, you can eliminate it. The fastest cure is to smell something or think about the smell of something awful. Carry around a bottle of camphor oil or eucalyptus oil. Take a deep whiff when tempted by the smell of something good. You can try other essential oils if these are too offensive to you. When you're without a bad smell try thinking of something disagreeable. Eventually the association will diminish, but it will never go away completely unless you completely give up eating the food that causes the trigger. Each time you eat the food—say popcorn for example—you will be training or conditioning your brain to crave the food when you smell or think of popcorn. If you never eat popcorn again, and use the camphor oil to eliminate this association, eventually the smell will fail to trigger cravings.

This is a powerful tool to re-train your behavior. Don't abuse it. Excessive use could lead to complete appetite suppression, resulting in devastating damage to your health. Food can become a habit. We eat without thinking at times. Breaking habits is sure a lot easier when food cravings are eliminated. You can change your schedule so that eating occurs at a different time. By making all new habits you can sometimes achieve better results. The previous example of using odors is just one way to re-train your behaviors. Many people have had success by changing the association of pleasure from eating the food to one of discomfort or pain. If you place a large rubber band on your wrist and every time you think about the bad habit, give it a snap, the association of pain eventually lessens the habit.

Remember, once you have eliminated the physical craving, all that remains is the habit.

Hypnosis and suggestion have also been used to change habits. They do help some people, but usually fail if the craving has not been treated, or the desire to quit is weak.

Activities that can assist in distracting you will help break habits. Try some of these, or make up your own.
Walking
Biking
Any exercise you enjoy
Wash your face in cold water
Phone a friend

I read once that to form a new habit takes three months, but to break an old one takes three years. I don't think it actually takes that long, it just seems that long. The **bible** has many references to 40 days as an important length of time. I suspect it takes about 40 days to form a new habit. If the new habit formed actually breaks some old habit then you have done both in only 40 days.

CHAPTER 20

TROUBLESHOOTING

GETTING RESULTS

If you have followed all the possible steps to cure your cravings, but you just don't get any lasting results, there are still further things to try. Be sure to check for diseases, or pathogens that may be the cause. Assuming otherwise good health, you may have trouble getting the proper nutrients into your brain. The problems can occur at several levels.

1. Inability to properly digest foods. You'll need digestive enzymes and possibly stomach acid supplements to correct this.

2. Inability to absorb nutrients. This can occur with parasites, fungal infection, bacterial overgrowth in the digestive tract, allergic reactions to dietary foods, lack of bile release, or failure of absorption—complexing factors. Here the solution is more complex. First eliminate pathogens and possible food irritants. Now stimulate bile by eating 2 tablespoons of olive oil with each meal. Chew your food and vitamin pills extra long to assist absorption in the mouth. Extensive testing to determine nutritional status may be required if these measures fail.

3. Your problem could be an inability to utilize nutrients after absorption. With food cravings, it is the brain that would be failing to receive or use the nutrients. The most common cause of poor circulation to the brain is arteriosclerosis. As the arteries feeding the brain clog and harden the circulation to the brain decreases, slowly reducing the available nutrients and impairing the ability of these nutrients to stop food cravings. Low blood pressure, or anemia can also have this effect.

To improve circulation to the brain try all of these:

1. Supplement at least 3 times daily with Ginkgo biloba extract. Also give yourself an extra dose whenever treating food cravings.

2. Supplement with cayenne capsules, on the same schedule as ginkgo.

3. Spend a few minutes on a slant board, with your head down. Try to start slowly and work up to longer times with this technique. Stop it if becomes uncomfortable.

4. Exercise vigorously for 30 minutes or more daily. The increased blood pressure improves circulation.

5. Drink seltzer water with your supplement. The carbonation increases permeability of the blood-brain barrier.

6. Cell membranes sometimes fail to function properly and nutrients don't get inside to do their job. Chelation may be necessary for some people, but requires a doctor's supervision. The following nutrients may help with this problem.

   MCT oil (medium chain triglycerides)
   Co – Enzyme Q10

Flax Oil
Potassium–Magnesium Aspartate
Thiamine
Malic Acid
Magnesium
Lipoic Acid
Pantothenic acid – B5

Hormones could be involved in your health problems. Testing can be very useful to identify the problem. These supplements often help if tests indicate a need:

1. DHEA
2. Thyroid hormone

Liver function could be the cause of your cravings. The liver is vital to health, and impaired liver function could be the cause of many cravings. If you crave sweets, candy especially, you could have bile troubles. If you are also constipated, and have light colored stools, along with digestive distress from fatty or fried foods, it is almost certain. You may require nutritional supplements to restore production and secretion of bile salts. If the gall bladder has been removed additional nutritional supplements may be required to restore health. A complete program should be developed with your health professional, to meet your individual needs.

Mineral deficiencies should always be suspected with any food craving. Taste tests as well as blood, hair and urine tests can reveal the problem. Zinc is only one common deficiency that can lead to inability to properly smell and taste food, leading to cravings. Complete testing is the fastest way to identify mineral imbalances, but a balanced supplement can be taken for a trial time (several months), and will often correct the problem.

RESTORING HEALTH PERMANENTLY

"WHEN HEALTH IS ABSENT, WISDOM CANNOT
REVEAL ITSELF, ART CANNOT BECOME MANIFEST,
STRENGTH CANNOT BE EXERTED, WEALTH
IS USELESS, AND REASON IS POWERLESS"
—*Herophilus 300 BC*

Cravings reveal just how powerless reason becomes when health is absent. Permanent elimination of cravings can only be maintained when health is restored.

The decline of our health usually begins with one or more of these problems:

1. Toxins accumulating faster than they are eliminated.

2. Nutritional factors that are inadequate or unbalanced.

3. Stress, either emotional or physical, including electro-magnetic and other environmental effects, that eventually overwhelms us.

These factors can trigger physical problems. Genetic and environmental factors will account for individual variation in just how well we can withstand those damages. Once a weakness occurs pathogens invade. They may be undetectable at first. These are the so called "subclinical" infections. They can influence cravings several ways.

Chronic low-grade infections, from viruses, bacteria, fungus, or parasites lower serotonin. These "bad bugs" produce toxins and your immune system battles them, also producing toxins. Eventually your body will increase its MAO, an enzyme you need to break down the toxic amines produced by the pathogens "bad bugs." As the level of MAO increases gradually it will have a bad side effect. MAO also breaks down serotonin, and other vital brain chemicals, depleting them. You need this MAO to breakdown toxic amines that cause high blood pressure and headaches, and, if amines get too high, strokes. But you also need your serotonin and other vital brain chemicals. Your body in its struggle to survive, identifies the biggest threat as toxic amines, and increases MAO. While the MAO does its job on the toxic amines, your brain chemicals suffer also.

To reduce these problems first you will need to identify the culprit or culprits. Chronic hidden infections can be cleaned up. The process involves improving your diet, regular exercise, sunshine, good hygiene and persistence. Any program should have these steps:
1. Identify and eliminate toxins
2. Improve nutrition (testing is important here)
3. Decrease stress
4. Kill pathogens

There are literally hundreds of safe effective foods, herbs, and nutritional supplements that will help. Individual symptoms and extensive questioning can reveal the best option for each person. Identifying the individual problem allows a more individual tailored program. Finding a good naturopath or herbalist to work with you will help.

Diet can also increase toxic amines. Certain foods are full of amines, forcing our body to increase MAO to deal with these foods. Common culprits are any fermented food, chocolate, cheese, summer sausage, salami, soy sauce, pickled herring, beer, wine, chicken livers, sour cream, fava beans, yogurt and all dairy products, avocados, raisins, ripe bananas, sauerkraut, caffeine, and most processed foods.

Food additives can also disturb serotonin and other brain chemicals. Avoid all processed foods, MSG, or hidden MSG (called hydrolyzed protein, among other names), aspartame (Nutra-sweet™ or Equal™), food dyes, coloring, bleaching agents, nitrites and nitrates.

Exercise is important in restoring health. Just walking 30 minutes a day outside in the sun if possible can make a world of difference. More vigorous

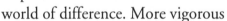

exercise, like running, will stimulate the brain's endorphins, giving you a "natural high" that lasts for about 30 minutes after running. These are zero calorie solutions that have helped many people fight food cravings. Unfortunately the runner's high that occurs with vigorous exercise only comes to conditioned athletes. You will need to stick to your exercise program to achieve this.

Vitamins and minerals can be vitally important to restoring chemical balance. Here again the best method is to test. Taste tests work fine for the minerals, zinc, potassium, magnesium, copper, chromium and manganese. You can obtain these "Chem. tests" from Bio-Science, *(see Sources)*. Other minerals can be tested with urine, blood, hair and saliva tests. If you don't want to test but would like to supplement your diet, the best advice is to take a mixture that has already been balanced to meet the needs of most people. By taking extra minerals you let your body take what it needs and to a certain extent it can balance its needs. It is only when one mineral is taken to excess that the system may not be able to compensate, and further imbalance occurs. Vitamins can also be consumed in a balanced mixture.

SOURCES

Most of the products mentioned in this book are available over the counter. No prescription is needed and supermarkets or health food stores often carry them. Even the hormone products are available as glandulars over the counter. A doctor's prescriptions are necessary if higher doses are required. Many health food stores will carry most if not all of these products. Some products like the "lite salt" mentioned under salt cravings are sold in supermarkets. Mail order is also an option.

Bio-Science
2398 Alaska Avenue
Port Orchard, WA 98366
Phone: (360) 871-1234
Orders: (800) 595-1089
Fax: (360) 871-6178

Barlean's Organic Oils
4936 Lake Terrell
Ferndale, WA 98248
Phone: (800) 445-3529

REFERENCES

1. The Amino Revolution by Robert Erdmann, Ph.D., with Meirion Jones, 1987

2. Fats That Can Save Your Life by Robert Erdmann, Ph.D., with Meirion Jones, 1990

3. J. Ethnophram,(90;30:265-279 & 90;30:281-294 & 90;30:295-305)

4. Int. J. Crude. Drug Res. 86;24 (Dec): 171-176

5. Metabolic Control and Disease by Philip Bondy, MD & Leon Rosenberg, MD 1980

6. The Pharmacological Basis of Therapeutics by Goodman and Gillman 1975

7. Textbook of Medical Physiology by Guyton 1986

8. Life Extension: a Practical Scientific Approach by Durk Pearson and Sandy Shaw 1982

9. Basic Neurochemistry by Raven Press, Editors

10. Neurobiology by Gordon Shepherd 1988

11. The Psychobiology of Obsessive-Compulsive Disorder by Zohar, Insel & Ramussen, editors 1991

12. Neurobiology of Taste and Smell by Thomas Finger & Wayne Silver, 1991

13. Improving your Child's Behavior Chemistry by Lendon Smith MD, 1977

14. Textbook of Endocrinology by Robert Williams, MD 1974

15. Your Body's Natural Wonder Drug, Melatonin by Russel Reiter and Jo Robinson, 1995

16. Does Aspartame Cause Human Brain Cancer? by HJ Roberts, MD, Journal of Advancement in Medicine, Vol. 4, No.4, Winter 1991

17. Aspartame: Is It Safe? by HJ Roberts, MD, Mastering Food Allergies, #61, Coeur d'Alene, Idaho

18. Repertory of the Homeopathic Materia Medica by J.T. Kent 1995 (reprint)

19. Herbally Yours by Penny C. Royal 1989

20. Townsend Letter for Doctors and Patients Dec 1995, pp 86-89

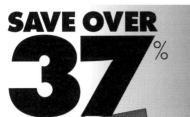
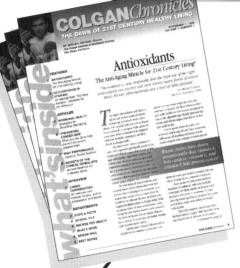